The Super Easy Keto Vegetarian Cookbook

Fast, Simple and Delicious Keto Vegetarian Recipes to Lose Weight and Feel Great

Dr. William Coleman

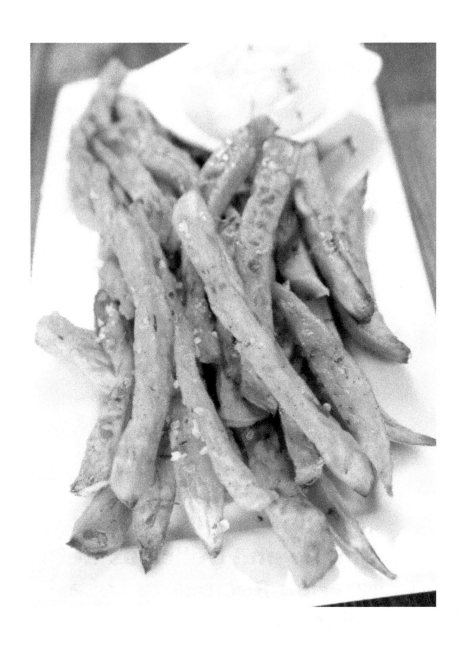

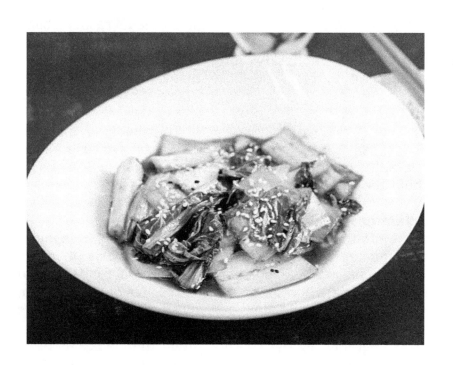

TABLE OF CONTENTS

INTRODUCTION

Essentially, a ketogenic diet is a diet that drastically restricts your carb intake and fat intake; this pushes your body to go into a state of ketosis.

Your body uses glucose from carbs to fuel metabolic pathways—meaning various bodily functions like digestion, breathing—essentially anything that needs energy. Glucose is therefore the primary pathway when it comes to sourcing the body's energy.

But the body has also another pathway, it can make use of fats to fuel the various bodily processes. And this is what is called ketosis. The body can only enter ketosis when there is no glucose available, thus the reason why eating a low-carb diet is essential in the keto diet.

Since no glucose is available, the body is pushed to use fats—it can either come from the food you consume or from your body's fat reserves—the adipose tissue or from the flabby parts of your body. This is how the keto diet helps you lose weight, by burning up all those stored fats that you have and using it to fuel bodily processes.

Ketosis is a very natural process, the body will soon adapt to this state and therefore you will be able to lose weight in no time but you will also become healthier and your physical and mental performances will improve. Your blood sugar levels will improve and you won't be predisposed to diabetes. Also, epilepsy and heart disease can be easily be prevented if you are on a ketogenic diet. Your cholesterol will improve and you will feel amazing in no time. How does that sound?

That said, if for whatever reason you are a vegetarian, following a ketogenic diet can be extremely difficult. A vegetarian diet is largely free of animal products, which means that food tends to be usually high in carbohydrates. Still, with careful planning, it is possible.

This Cookbook will provide you with various easy and delicious dishes to help you stick to your ketogenic diet plan while being a vegetarian.

Enjoy!

Almond Cinnamon Smoothie

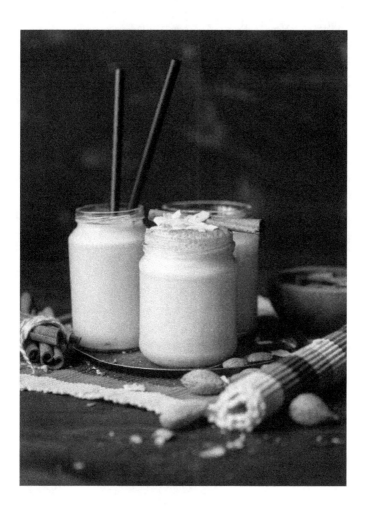

Preparation Time: 10 minutes

Servings: 1

Ingredients:

- ¾ cup almond milk, unsweetened
- ¼ cup coconut oil
- 1 tablespoon almond butter, unsweetened
- 1 tablespoon vanilla protein powder
- 1/8 teaspoon cinnamon

Directions:

1. Add into your blender all the ingredients, blend them until they are nice and smooth. Serve and enjoy!

Nutritional Values (Per Serving):

Calories: 500 Fat: 43 g Carbohydrates: 10 g Sugar: 2 g Protein: 14.6 g Cholesterol: 0 mg

Bulletproof Coffee

Preparation Time: 3 minutes

Serving: 2

Ingredients:

- 2 ½ heaping tbsp. ground bulletproof coffee beans
- 1 cup water
- 1 tbsp MCT oil
- 2 tbsp unsalted butter

Directions:

1. Using a coffee maker, brew one cup of coffee with the ground coffee beans and water.
2. Transfer the coffee to a blender and add the MCT oil and butter. Blend the mixture until frothy and smooth.
3. Divide the drink into two teacups and enjoy immediately.

Nutrition:

Calories:64, Total Fat:7.3 g, Saturated Fat: 5.3g, Total Carbs:3 g, Dietary Fiber: 2g, Sugar: 2g, Protein: 3g, Sodium: 300mg

Eggplant and Peppers Soup

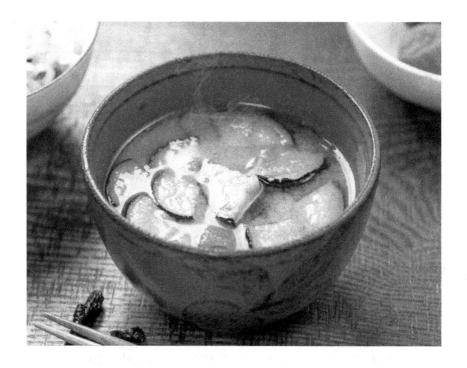

Preparation time: 10 minutes

Cooking time: 40 minutes

Servings: 4

Ingredients:

- 2 red bell peppers, chopped
- 3 scallions, chopped
- 3 garlic cloves, minced

- 2 tablespoon olive oil
- Salt and black pepper to the taste
- 5 cups vegetable stock
- 1 bay leaf
- ½ cup coconut cream
- 1 pound eggplants, roughly cubed
- 2 tablespoons basil, chopped

Directions:

1. Heat up a pot with the oil over medium heat, add the scallions and the garlic and sauté for 5 minutes.
2. Add the peppers and the eggplants and sauté for 5 minutes more.
3. Add the remaining ingredients, toss, bring to a simmer, cook for 30 minutes, ladle into bowls and serve for lunch.

Nutrition:

calories 180, fat 2, fiber 3, carbs 5, protein 10

Roasted Cauliflower and Broccoli

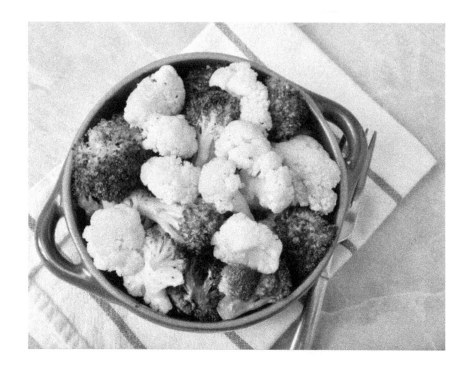

Preparation Time: 10 minutes

Cooking Time: 15 minutes

Servings: 12

Ingredients:

- 4 cups broccoli, florets
- 4 cups cauliflower, florets
- 6 cloves garlic, minced

- 2/3 cup Parmesan cheese, grated, divided
- 1/3 cup extra-virgin olive oil
- Pepper and salt to taste

Directions:

1. Preheat your oven to 450° Fahrenheit.
2. Spray with cooking spray a baking dish, then set it aside.
3. Add broccoli, cauliflower, half of the cheese, garlic, and olive oil into a mixing bowl and toss well to blend.
4. Season with salt and pepper.
5. Arrange cauliflower and broccoli mixture in your prepared baking dish.
6. Bake for 15 minutes in preheated oven.
7. Just before serving add remaining cheese on top.
8. Serve hot and enjoy!

Nutritional Values (Per Serving):

Calories: 81 Carbohydrates: 3.1 G Fat: 6.7 G Sugar: 1.1 G Cholesterol: 5 Mg Protein: 1.9 G

Keto Caesar Salad

Preparation Time: 15 minutes

Servings: 8

Ingredients:

- 8 cups romaine lettuce, chopped
- 2 tablespoons lemon juice, fresh
- ¼ cup Parmesan cheese, grated, fresh
- ¼ teaspoon garlic powder
- 1 tablespoon mayonnaise
- ¼ cup extra-virgin olive oil
- ¼ teaspoon pepper

Directions:

1. In mixing bowl, combine olive oil, garlic powder, lemon juice and mayonnaise. Add lettuce and cheese to the bowl. Season with pepper.
2. Cover bowl and place in the fridge for about an hour.
3. Just before serving toss salad and enjoy!

Nutritional Values (Per Serving):

Calories: 102 Fat: 9.3 g Sugar: 0.8 g Cholesterol: 5 mg Carbohydrates: 2.3 g Protein: 3.3 g

Vietnamese "Vermicelli" Salad

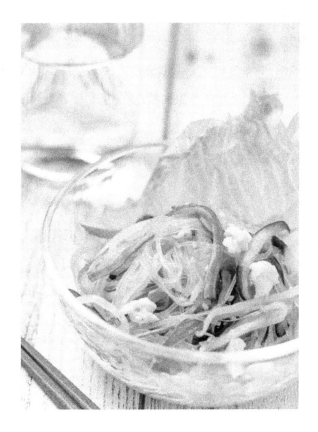

Preparation Time: 5 min

Cooking Time: Serves: 4

Ingredients:

- 100 grams Carrot, sliced into thin strips
- 200 grams Cucumbers, spiralized

- 2 tbsp Roasted Peanuts, roughly chopped
- ¼ cup Fresh Mint, chopped
- ¼ cup Fresh Cilantro, chopped
- 1 tbsp Stevia
- 2 tbsp Fresh Lime Juice
- tbsp Vegan Fish Sauce
- 2 cloves Garlic, minced
- 1 Green Chili, deseeded and minced
- 2 tbsp Sesame Oil

Directions:

1. Whisk together sugar, lime juice, sesame oil, fish sauce, minced garlic, and chopped chili. Set aside.
2. In a bowl, toss together cucumbers, carrots, cucumbers, peanuts, mint, cilantro, and prepared dressing.
3. Serve chilled.

Nutritional Values:

Kcal per serve: 249 Fat: 11 g. Protein: 5 g. Carbs: 8 g.

Cajun Tofu in Mushrooms

Preparation Time: 10 minutes

Cooking Time: 43 minutes

Serving: 4

Ingredients:

- 2 tbsp olive oil
- ½ celery stalk, chopped
- 1 small red onion, finely chopped
- 1 lb tofu, pressed and crumbled
- Salt and black pepper to taste
- 2 tbsp mayonnaise
- 1 tsp Cajun seasoning
- ½ tsp garlic powder
- ½ cup shredded Gouda cheese
- 2 large eggs
- 4 large caps Portobello mushrooms
- 1 tbsp almond meal
- 2 tbsp shredded Parmesan cheese
- 1 tbsp chopped fresh parsley

Directions:

1. Preheat the oven to 350 F and lightly grease a baking sheet with cooking spray. Set aside.

2. Heat half of the olive oil in a medium skillet over medium heat and sauté the celery, red onion until softened, 3 minutes. Transfer to a medium mixing bowl.

3. Add the remaining olive oil to the skillet, season the tofu with salt, black pepper, and cook until brown, 10 minutes. Turn the heat off and transfer to the same bowl.

4. Pour in the mayonnaise, Cajun seasoning, garlic powder, Gouda cheese, and crack in the eggs. Mix well.

5. Arrange the mushrooms on the baking sheet and fill with the tofu mix.

6. In a small bowl, mix the almond meal, Parmesan cheese, and sprinkle on top of the mushroom filling. Cover with foil and bake in the oven until the cheese melts, 30 minutes.

7. Remove the stuffed mushrooms, take off the foil, and garnish with the parsley.

8. Serve immediately.

Nutrition:

Calories: 400, Total Fat: 29.1g, Saturated Fat: 8.1g, Total Carbs: 10 g, Dietary Fiber:3 g, Sugar: 2g, Protein:29 g, Sodium: 414mg

Creamy Cabbage with Tofu and Pine Nuts

Preparation Time: 5 minutes

Cooking Time: 20 minutes

Serving: 4

Ingredients:

For the fried tofu:

- 2 tbsp butter
- 25 oz tofu, cut into 6 slabs

For the creamy cabbage:

- 2 oz butter
- 25 oz green canon cabbage, shredded
- 1 ¼ cups heavy cream
- ½ cup chopped fresh marjoram
- Salt and black pepper to taste
- ½ lemon, zested
- 2 tbsp toasted pine nuts

Directions:

For the fried tofu:

1. Melt the butter in a medium skillet over medium heat and fry the tofu on both sides until lightly

brown on the outside, 10 minutes. Transfer to a plate and keep warm until ready to serve.

For the creamy cabbage:

2. Melt the butter in the skillet and sauté the cabbage while occasionally stirring until the cabbage turns golden brown, 4 minutes.
3. Mix in the heavy cream, allow bubbling, and season with the marjoram, salt, black pepper, and lemon zest.
4. Divide the tofu onto four plates, spoon the cabbage to the side of the tofu, and sprinkle the pine nuts on the cabbage.
5. Serve warm.

Nutrition:

Calories:269, Total Fat: 21.6g, Saturated Fat: 7.8g, Total Carbs: 6g, Dietary Fiber: 1g, Sugar: 3g, Protein: 13g, Sodium: 298mg

Avocado Coconut Pie

Preparation Time: 30 minutes

Cooking Time: 50 minutes

Serving: 4

Ingredients:

For the piecrust:

- 1 tbsp flax seed powder + 3 tbsp water
- 4 tbsp coconut flour
- 4 tbsp chia seeds
- ¾ cup almond flour
- 1 tbsp psyllium husk powder
- 1 tsp baking powder
- 1 pinch salt
- 3 tbsp coconut oil
- 4 tbsp water

For the filling:

- 2 ripe avocados
- 1 cup vegan mayonnaise
- 3 tbsp flax seed powder + 9 tbsp water
- 2 tbsp fresh parsley, finely chopped
- 1 jalapeno, finely chopped

- ½ tsp onion powder
- ¼ tsp salt
- ½ cup cashew cream
- 1¼ cups shredded tofu cheese

Directions:

1. In 2 separate bowls, mix the different portions of flax seed powder with the respective quantity of water. Allow absorbing for 5 minutes.
2. Preheat the oven to 350 F.
3. In a food processor, add the coconut flour, chia seeds, almond flour, psyllium husk powder, baking powder, salt, coconut oil, water, and the smaller portion of the flax egg. Blend the Ingredients until the resulting dough forms into a ball.
4. Line a spring form pan with about 12-inch diameter of parchment paper and spread the dough in the pan. Bake for 10 to 15 minutes or until a light golden brown color is achieved.
5. Meanwhile, cut the avocado into halves lengthwise, remove the pit, and chop the pulp.

6. Put in a bowl and add the mayonnaise, remaining flax egg, parsley, jalapeno, onion powder, salt, cashew cream, and tofu cheese. Combine well.
7. Remove the piecrust when ready and fill with the creamy mixture. Level the filling with a spatula and continue baking for 35 minutes or until lightly golden brown.
8. When ready, take out. Cool before slicing and serving with a baby spinach salad.

Nutrition:

Calories:680, Total Fat:71.8 g, Saturated Fat:20.9 g, Total Carbs: 10g, Dietary Fiber:7 g, Sugar: 2g, Protein: 3g, Sodium:525 mg

Peppers and Celery Sauté

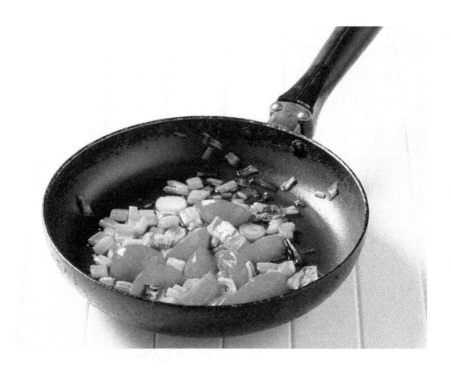

Preparation time: 10 minutes

Cooking time: 15 minutes

Servings: 4

Ingredients:

- 1 red bell pepper, cut into medium chunks
- 1 green bell pepper, cut into medium chunks
- 1 celery stalk, chopped

- 2 scallions, chopped
- 2 tablespoons olive oil
- Salt and black pepper to the taste
- 1 tablespoons parsley, chopped
- 1 teaspoon cumin, ground
- 2 garlic cloves, minced

Directions:

1. Heat up a pan with the oil over medium heat, add the scallions, garlic and cumin and sauté for 5 minutes.
2. Add the peppers, celery and the other ingredients, toss, cook over medium heat for 10 minutes more, divide between plates and serve.

Nutrition:

calories 87, fat 2.4, fiber 3, carbs 5, protein 4

Sweet Potatoes Side Dish

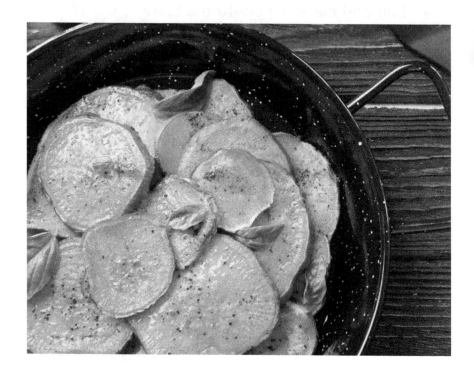

Preparation time: 10 minutes

Cooking time: 3 hours

Servings: 10

Ingredients:

- 4 pounds sweet potatoes, thinly sliced
- 3 tablespoons stevia
- ½ cup orange juice

- A pinch of salt and black pepper
- ½ teaspoon thyme, dried
- ½ teaspoon sage, dried
- 2 tablespoons olive oil

Directions:

1. Arrange potato slices on the bottom of your slow cooker.
2. In a bowl, mix orange juice with salt, pepper, stevia, thyme, sage and oil and whisk well.
3. Add this over potatoes, cover slow cooker and cook on High for 3 hours.
4. Divide between plates and serve as a side dish.
5. Enjoy!

Nutrition:

calories 189, fat 4, fiber 4, carbs 36, protein 4

Rustic Mashed Potatoes

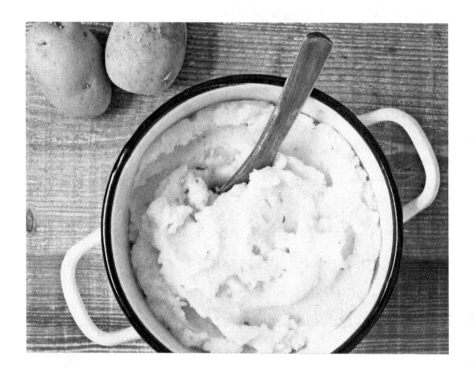

Preparation time: 10 minutes

Cooking time: 4 hours

Servings: 6

Ingredients:

- 6 garlic cloves, peeled
- 3 pounds gold potatoes, peeled and cubed
- 1 bay leaf

- 1 cup coconut milk
- 28 ounces veggie stock
- 3 tablespoons olive oil
- Salt and black pepper to the taste

Directions:

1. In your slow cooker, mix potatoes with stock, bay leaf, garlic, salt and pepper, cover and cook on High for 4 hours.
2. Drain potatoes and garlic, return them to your slow cooker and mash using a potato masher.
3. Add oil and coconut milk, whisk well, divide between plates and serve as a side dish.
4. Enjoy!

Nutrition:

calories 135, fat 5, fiber 1, carbs 20, protein 3

Beets And Carrots

Preparation time: 10 minutes

Cooking time: 7 hours

Servings: 8

Ingredients:

- 2 tablespoons stevia
- ¾ cup pomegranate juice
- 2 teaspoons ginger, grated
- 2 and ½ pounds beets, peeled and cut into wedges
- 12 ounces carrots, cut into medium wedges

Directions:

1. In your slow cooker, mix beets with carrots, ginger, stevia and pomegranate juice, toss, cover and cook on Low for 7 hours.
2. Divide between plates and serve as a side dish.
3. Enjoy!

Nutrition:

calories 125, fat 0, fiber 4, carbs 28, protein 3

Creamy Corn

Preparation time: 10 minutes

Cooking time: 3 hours

Servings: 6

Ingredients:

- 50 ounces corn
- 1 cup almond milk
- 1 tablespoon stevia
- 8 ounces coconut cream
- A pinch of white pepper

Directions:

1. In your slow cooker, mix corn with almond milk, stevia, cream and white pepper, toss, cover and cook on High for 3 hours.
2. Divide between plates and serve as a side dish.
3. Enjoy!

Nutrition:

calories 200, fat 5, fiber 7, carbs 12, protein 4

Minted Peas

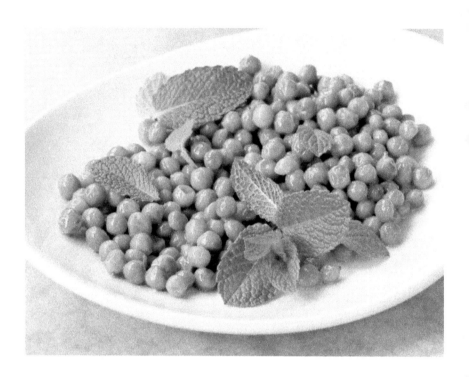

Preparation time: 5 minutes

cooking time: 5 minutes

servings: 4

Ingredients

- 1 tablespoon olive oil
- 4 cups peas, fresh or frozen (not canned
- ½ teaspoon sea salt

- freshly ground black pepper
- 3 tablespoons chopped fresh mint

Directions

1. In a large sauté pan, heat the olive oil over medium-high heat until hot. Add the peas and cook, about 5 minutes.
2. Remove the pan from heat. Stir in the salt, season with pepper, and stir in the mint.
3. Serve hot.

Edamame Donburi

Preparation time: 5 minutes

cooking time: 20 minutes

servings: 4

Ingredients

- 1 cup fresh or frozen shelled edamame
- 1 tablespoon canola or grapeseed oil
- 1 medium yellow onion, minced
- 5 shiitake mushroom caps, lightly rinsed, patted dry, and cut into 1/4-inch strips
- 1 teaspoon grated fresh ginger
- 3 green onions, minced
- 8 ounces firm tofu, drained and crumbled
- 2 tablespoons soy sauce
- 3 cups hot cooked white or brown rice
- 1 tablespoon toasted sesame oil
- 1 tablespoon toasted sesame seeds, for garnish

Directions

1. In a small saucepan of boiling salted water, cook the edamame until tender, about 10 minutes.

Drain and set aside.

2. In a large skillet, heat the canola oil over medium heat. Add the onion, cover, and cook until softened, about 5 minutes.

3. Add the mushrooms and cook, uncovered, 5 minutes longer. Stir in the ginger and green onions.

4. Add the tofu and soy sauce and cook until heated through, stirring to combine well, about 5 minutes.

5. Stir in the cooked edamame and cook until heated through, about 5 minutes.

6. Divide the hot rice among 4 bowls, top each with the edamame and tofu mixture, and drizzle on the sesame oil.

7. Sprinkle with sesame seeds and serve immediately.

Sicilian Stuffed Tomatoes

Preparation time: 10 minutes

cooking time: 30 minutes

servings: 4

Ingredients

- 2 cups water
- 1 cup couscous
- Salt
- 3 green onions, minced
- 1/3 cup golden raisins
- 1 teaspoon finely grated orange zest
- 4 large ripe tomatoes
- 1/3 cup toasted pine nuts
- 1/4 cup minced fresh parsley
- Freshly ground black pepper
- 2 teaspoons olive oil

Directions

1. Preheat the oven to 375°F. Lightly oil a 9 x 13-inch baking pan and set aside. In a large saucepan, bring the water to a boil over high

heat. Stir in the couscous and salt to taste and remove from the heat. Stir in the green onions, raisins, and orange zest. Cover and set aside for 5 minutes.

2. Cut a 1/2-inch-thick slice off the top of each of the tomatoes. Scoop out the pulp, keeping the tomato shells intact. Chop the pulp and place it in a large bowl. Add the couscous mixture along with the pine nuts, parsley, and salt and pepper to taste. Mix well.

3. Fill the tomatoes with the mixture and place them in the prepared pan. Drizzle the tomatoes with the oil, cover with foil, and bake until hot, about 20 minutes.

4. Serve immediately.

Popovers

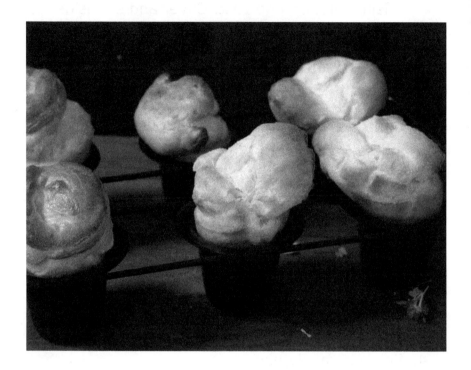

Preparation Time: 5 mins

Servings: 6

Ingredients:

- 4 egg whites
- 1 c. All-purpose flour
- 1 c. fat-free milk
- ¼ tsp. salt

Directions:

1. Preheat your oven to 425 0F.
2. Coat a six cup metal or glass muffin mold with cooking spray and heat the mold in the oven for two minutes.
3. In a bowl, add the flour, milk, salt, and egg whites. Use a mixer to beat until it's smooth.
4. Fill the heated molds two-thirds of the way full.
5. Bake until the muffins are golden brown and puffy, around half an hour.
6. Serve.

Nutrition:

Calories: 101, Fat:0 g, Carbs:18 g, Protein:6 g, Sugars:2 g, Sodium:125 mg

Cinnamon-Scented Quinoa

Preparation Time: 5 mins

Servings: 4

Ingredients:

- Chopped walnuts
- 1 ½ c. water
- Maple syrup
- 2 cinnamon sticks
- 1 c. quinoa

Directions:

1. Add the quinoa to a bowl and wash it in several changes of water until the water is clear. When washing quinoa, rub grains and allow them to settle before you pour off the water.
2. Use a large fine-mesh sieve to drain the quinoa. Prepare your pressure cooker with a trivet and steaming basket. Place the quinoa and the cinnamon sticks in the basket and pour the water.
3. Close and lock the lid. Cook at high pressure for

6 minutes. When the cooking time is up, release the pressure using the quick release method.

4. Fluff the quinoa with a fork and remove the cinnamon sticks. Divide the cooked quinoa among serving bowls and top with maple syrup and chopped walnuts.

Nutrition:

Calories: 160, Fat:3 g, Carbs:28 g, Protein:6 g, Sugars:19 g, Sodium:40 mg

Broccoli Stew

Preparation time: 10 minutes

Cooking time: 40 minutes

Servings: 4

Ingredients:

- 1 broccoli head, separated into florets
- 2 teaspoons coriander seeds
- A drizzle of olive oil
- 1 onion, peeled and chopped
- Salt and ground black pepper, to taste
- A pinch of red pepper, crushed
- 1 small ginger piece, peeled, and chopped
- 1 garlic clove, peeled and minced
- 28 ounces canned pureed tomatoes

Directions:

1. Put water in a pot, add the salt, bring to a boil over medium-high heat, add the broccoli florets, steam them for 2 minutes, transfer them to a bowl filled with ice water, drain them, and leave aside.

2. Heat up a pan over medium-high heat, add the coriander seeds, toast them for 4 minutes, transfer to a grinder, ground them, and set aside as well.
3. Heat up a pot with the oil over medium heat, add the onions, salt, pepper, and red pepper, stir, and cook for 7 minutes.
4. Add the ginger, garlic, and coriander seeds, stir, and cook for 3 minutes.
5. Add the tomatoes, bring to a boil, and simmer for 10 minutes.
6. Add the broccoli, stir and cook the stew for 12 minutes.
7. Divide into bowls and serve.

Nutrition:

Calories - 150, Fat - 4, Fiber - 2, Carbs - 5, Protein - 12

Bok Choy Stir-fry

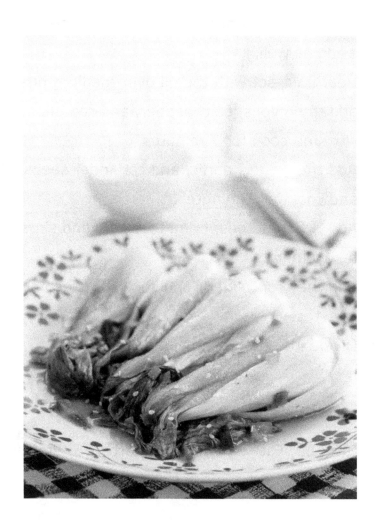

Preparation time: 10 minutes

Cooking time: 7 minutes

Servings: 2

Ingredients:

- 2 garlic cloves, peeled and minced
- 2 cup bok choy, chopped
- 2 bacon slices, chopped
- Salt and ground black pepper, to taste
- A drizzle of avocado oil

Directions:

1. Heat up a pan with the oil over medium heat, add the bacon, stir, and brown until crispy, transfer to paper towels, and drain the grease.
2. Return the pan to medium heat, add the garlic and bok choy, stir, and cook for 4 minutes.
3. Add the salt, pepper, and return the bacon to the pan, stir, cook for 1 minute, divide on plates, and serve.

Nutrition:

Calories - 50, Fat - 1, Fiber - 1, Carbs - 2, Protein - 2

Sautéed Mustard Greens

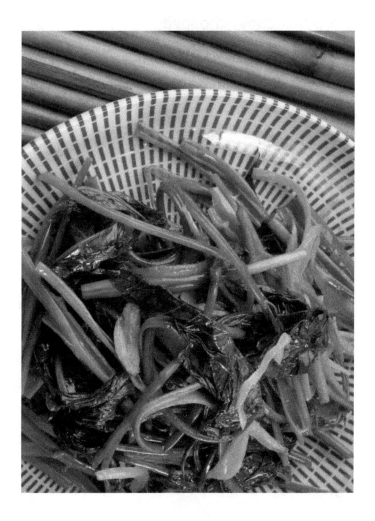

Preparation time: 5 minutes

Cooking time: 15 minutes

Servings: 4

Ingredients:

- 2 garlic cloves, peeled and minced
- 1 pound mustard greens, torn
- 1 tablespoon olive oil
- ½ cup onion, sliced
- Salt and ground black pepper, to taste
- 3 tablespoons vegetable stock
- ¼ teaspoon dark sesame oil

Directions:

1. Heat up a pan with the oil over medium heat, add the onions, stir, and brown them for 10 minutes.
2. Add the garlic, stir, and cook for 1 minute.
3. Add the stock, greens, salt, and pepper, stir, and cook for 5 minutes.
4. Add more salt and pepper, and sesame oil, toss to coat, divide on plates, and serve.

Nutrition:

Calories - 120, Fat - 3, Fiber - 1, Carbs - 3, Protein - 6

Mustard Greens and Spinach Soup

Preparation time: 10 minutes

Cooking time: 15 minutes

Servings: 6

Ingredients:

- ½ teaspoon fenugreek seeds
- 1 teaspoon cumin seeds
- 1 tablespoon avocado oil
- 1 teaspoon coriander seeds
- 1 cup onion, chopped
- 1 tablespoon garlic, minced
- 1 tablespoon fresh ginger, grated
- ½ teaspoon turmeric
- 5 cups mustard greens, chopped
- 3 cups coconut milk
- 1 tablespoon jalapeño, chopped
- 5 cups spinach, torn
- Salt and ground black pepper, to taste
- 2 teaspoons butter
- ½ teaspoon paprika

Directions:

1. Heat up a pot with the oil over medium-high heat, add the coriander, fenugreek, and cumin seeds, stir, and brown them for 2 minutes.
2. Add the onions, stir, and cook for 3 minutes. Add the half of the garlic, jalapeños, ginger, and turmeric, stir, and cook for 3 minutes.
3. Add the mustard greens, and spinach, stir, and sauté everything for 10 minutes.
4. Add the milk, salt, and pepper, and blend the soup using an immersion blender.
5. Heat up a pan with the butter over medium heat, add the garlic, and paprika, stir well, and take off the heat.
6. Heat up the soup over medium heat, ladle into soup bowls, drizzle with butter and sprinkle with paprika all over, and serve.

Nutrition:

Calories - 143, Fat - 6, Fiber - 3, Carbs - 7, Protein - 7

Catalan-style Greens

Preparation time: 10 minutes

Cooking time: 15 minutes

Servings: 4

Ingredients:

- 1 apple, cored and chopped
- 1 onion, peeled and sliced
- 3 tablespoons avocado oil
- ¼ cup raisins
- 6 garlic cloves, peeled and chopped
- ¼ cup pine nuts, toasted
- ¼ cup balsamic vinegar
- 2½ cups Swiss chard
- 2½ cups spinach, and
- Salt and ground black pepper, to taste
- A pinch of nutmeg

Directions:

1. Heat up a pan with the oil over medium-high heat, add the onion, stir, and cook for 3 minutes.

2. Add the apple, stir, and cook for 4 minutes.

3. Add the garlic, stir, and cook for 1 minute.

4. Add the raisins, vinegar, spinach, and chard, stir, and cook for 5 minutes.

5. Add the nutmeg, salt, and pepper, stir, cook for a few seconds, divide on plates, and serve.

Nutrition:

Calories - 120, Fat - 1, Fiber - 2, Carbs - 3, Protein - 6

Root Vegetable Bisque

Preparation time: 5 minutes

cooking time: 35 minutes

servings: 4 to 6

Ingredients

- 1 tablespoon olive oil
- 3 large shallots, chopped
- 2 large carrots, shredded
- 2 medium parsnips, shredded
- 1 medium potato, peeled and chopped
- 2 garlic cloves, minced
- 1/2 teaspoon dried thyme
- 1/4 teaspoon dried marjoram
- 4 cups vegetable broth, homemade (see Light Vegetable Broth or store-bought, or water
- 1 cup plain unsweetened soy milk
- Salt and freshly ground black pepper
- 1 tablespoon minced fresh parsley, garnish

Directions

1. In a large soup pot, heat the oil over medium heat. Add the shallots, carrots, parsnips, potato, and garlic. Cover and cook until softened, about 5 minutes.

2. Add the thyme, marjoram, and broth and bring to a boil. Reduce heat to low and simmer, uncovered, until the vegetables are tender, about 30 minutes.

3. Puree the soup in the pot with an immersion blender or in a blender or food processor in batches if necessary, then return to the pot.

4. Stir in the soy milk and taste, adjusting seasonings if necessary.

5. Heat the soup over low heat until hot. Ladle into bowls, sprinkle with parsley, and serve.

Curried Pumpkin Soup

Preparation time: 5 minutes

cooking time: 22 minutes

servings: 4 to 6

Ingredients

- 1 tablespoon olive oil
- 1 medium onion, chopped
- 1 garlic clove, minced
- 1 teaspoon grated fresh ginger
- 1 tablespoon hot or mild curry powder
- 1 (16-ouncecan pumpkin puree or 2 cups cooked fresh pumpkin
- 3 cups vegetable broth, homemade (see Light Vegetable Broth or store-bought, or water
- Salt
- 1 (13.5-ouncecan unsweetened coconut milk
- 1 tablespoon minced fresh parsley, for garnish
- Mango chutney, for garnish (optional
- Chopped roasted cashews, for garnish (optional)

Directions

1. In a large soup pot, heat the oil over medium heat. Add the onion and garlic and cover and cook until softened, about 7 minutes. Stir in the ginger, curry powder, and cook for 30 seconds over low heat, stirring constantly.

2. Stir in the pumpkin, broth, and salt to taste and bring to a boil. Reduce heat to low, cover, and simmer, uncovered, until the flavors are blended, about 15 minutes.

3. Use an immersion blender to puree the soup in the pot or transfer in batches to a blender or food processor, puree, then return to the pot, and season with salt and pepper to taste. Add coconut milk and heat until hot.

4. Ladle into soup bowls, sprinkle with parsley and a spoonful of chutney sprinkled with chopped cashews, if using, and serve.

Cream of Tomato Soup

Preparation Time: 5 Minutes

Cooking Time: 5 Minutes

Servings:2

Ingredients

- 1 (28-ounce) can crushed, diced, or whole peeled tomatoes, undrained
- 1 to 2 teaspoons dried herbs
- 2 to 3 teaspoons onion powder (optional)
- ¾ to 1 cup unsweetened nondairy milk
- ½ teaspoon salt, or to taste
- Freshly ground black pepper

Directions

1. Preparing the Ingredients.
2. Pour the tomatoes and their juices into a large pot and bring them to near-boiling over medium heat.
3. Add the dried herbs, onion powder (if using), milk, salt, and pepper to taste. Stir to combine. If you used diced or whole tomatoes, use a hand

blender to purée the soup until smooth. (Alternatively, let the soup cool for a few minutes, then transfer to a countertop blender.)

4. Leftovers will keep in an airtight container for up to 1 week in the refrigerator or up to 1 month in the freezer (though if you want leftovers for this soup, you might want to double the recipe).

Per Serving (2 cups)

Calories: 90; Protein: 4g; Total fat: 3g; Saturated fat: 0g; Carbohydrates: 16g; Fiber: 4g

Spicy Black Bean Orzo Soup

Preparation Time: 5 Minutes

Cooking Time: 50 Minutes

Servings:4 To 6

Ingredients

- 2 tablespoons olive oil
- 3 garlic cloves, minced
- 1 tablespoon chili powder
- 1 teaspoon dried oregano
- 41/2 cups cooked or 3 (15.5-ounce) cans black beans, drained and rinsed
- 1 small jalapeño, seeded and finely chopped (optional)
- 1/4 cup minced oil-packed sun-dried tomatoes
- 4 cups vegetable broth, homemade (see Light Vegetable Broth) or store-bought, or water
- 1 cup water
- Salt and freshly ground black pepper
- 1/2 cup orzo
- 2 tablespoons chopped fresh cilantro, for garnish

Directions

1. In a large soup pot, heat the oil over medium heat. Add the garlic and cook until fragrant, about 1 minute. Stir in the chili powder, oregano, beans, jalapeño, if using, tomatoes, broth, water, and salt and pepper to taste. Simmer for 30 minutes to blend flavors.

2. Puree the soup in the pot with an immersion blender or in a blender or food processor, in batches if necessary, and return to the pot. Cook the soup 15 minutes longer over medium heat. Taste, adjusting seasonings, and add more water if necessary.

3. While the soup is simmering, cook the orzo in a pot of boiling salted water, stirring occasionally, until al dente, about 5 minutes. Drain the orzo and divide it among the soup bowls. Ladle the soup into the bowls, garnish with cilantro, and serve.

Creamy Tofu with Green Beans and Keto Fettuccine

Preparation Time: 40 minutes + overtime chilling time

Serving size: 4

Ingredients:

For the keto fettuccine:

- 1 cup shredded mozzarella cheese
- 1 egg yolk

For the creamy tofu and green beans:

- 1 tbsp olive oil
- 4 tofu, cut into thin strips
- Salt and black pepper to taste
- ½ cup green beans, chopped
- 1 lemon, zested and juiced
- ¼ cup vegetable broth
- 1 cup plain yogurt
- 6 basil leaves, chopped
- 1 cup shaved parmesan cheese for topping

Directions:

For the keto fettucine:

1. Pour the cheese into a medium safe-microwave bowl and melt in the microwave for 35 minutes or until melted.
2. Take out the bowl and allow cooling for 1 minute only to warm the cheese but not cool completely. Mix in the egg yolk until well-combined.
3. Lay a parchment paper on a flat surface, pour the cheese mixture on top and cover with another parchment paper. Using a rolling pin, flatten the dough into 1/8-inch thickness.
4. Take off the parchment paper and cut the dough into thick fettuccine strands. Place in a bowl and refrigerate overnight.
5. When ready to cook, bring 2 cups of water to a boil in medium saucepan and add the keto fettuccine. Cook for 40 seconds to 1 minute and then drain through a colander. Run cold water over the pasta and set aside to cool.

For the creamy tofu and green beans:

6. Heat the olive oil in a large skillet, season the tofu with salt, black pepper, and cook in the oil

until brown on the outside and slightly cooked through, 10 minutes.

7. Mix in the green beans and cook until softened, 5 minutes.

8. Stir in the lemon zest, lemon juice, and vegetable broth. Cook for 5 more minutes or until the liquid reduces by a quarter.

9. Add the plain yogurt and mix well. Pour in the keto fettuccine and basil, fold in well and cook for 1 minute. Adjust the taste with salt and black pepper as desired.

10. Dish the food onto serving plates, top with the parmesan cheese and serve warm.

Nutrition:

Calories:721, Total Fat:76.8g, Saturated Fat:21.2g, Total Carbs:2g, Dietary Fiber:0g, Sugar:0g, Protein:9g, Sodium:309mg

Yellow Mung Bean Salad With Broccoli And Mango

Preparation Time: 5 Minutes

Cooking Time: 20 Minutes

Servings:4

Ingredients

- 1/2 cup yellow mung beans, picked over, rinsed, and drained
- 3 cups small broccoli florets, blanched
- 1 ripe mango, peeled, pitted, and chopped
- 1 small red bell pepper, chopped
- 1 jalapeño or other hot green chile, seeded and minced
- 2 tablespoons chopped fresh cilantro
- 1 teaspoon grated fresh ginger
- 2 tablespoons fresh lemon juice
- 3 tablespoons grapeseed oil
- 1/3 cup unsalted roasted cashews, for garnish

Directions

1. In a saucepan of boiling salted water, cook the

mung beans until just tender, 18 to 20 minutes. Drain and run under cold water to cool.

2. Transfer the beans to a large bowl. Add the broccoli, mango, bell pepper, chile, and cilantro.

3. Set aside.

4. In a small bowl, combine the ginger, lemon juice, oil.

5. Stir to mix well, then pour the dressing over the vegetables and toss to combine.

6. Sprinkle with cashews and serve.

Cranberry-Carrot Salad

Preparation Time: 15 Minutes

Cooking Time: 0 Minutes

Servings:4

Ingredients

- 1 pound carrots, shredded
- 1 cup sweetened dried cranberries
- 1/2 cup toasted walnut pieces
- 2 tablespoons fresh lemon juice
- 3 tablespoons toasted walnut oil
- 1/8 teaspoon freshly ground black pepper

Directions

1. In a large bowl, combine the carrots, cranberries, and walnuts. Set aside.
2. In a small bowl, whisk together the lemon juice, walnut oil and pepper. Pour the dressing over the salad, toss gently to combine and serve.

Apple-Sunflower Spinach Salad

Preparation Time: 5 Minutes

Cooking Time: 0 Minutes

Servings:1

Ingredients

- 1 cup baby spinach
- ½ apple, cored and chopped
- ¼ red onion, thinly sliced (optional)
- 2 tablespoons sunflower seeds or Cinnamon-Lime Sunflower Seeds
- 2 tablespoons dried cranberries
- 2 tablespoons Raspberry Vinaigrette

Directions

1. Arrange the spinach on a plate. Top with the apple, red onion (if using), sunflower seeds, and cranberries, and drizzle with the vinaigrette.

Nutrition Per Serving

Calories: 444; Protein: 7g; Total fat: 28g; Saturated fat: 3g; Carbohydrates: 53g; Fiber: 8g

Sunshine Fiesta Salad

Preparation Time: 15 Minutes

Cooking Time: 0 Minutes

Servings:4

Ingredients

For The Vinaigrette

- Juice of 2 limes
- 1 tablespoon olive oil
- 1 tablespoon maple syrup or agave
- ¼ teaspoon sea salt

For The Salad

- 2 cups cooked quinoa
- 1 tablespoon Taco Seasoning or store-bought taco seasoning
- 2 heads romaine lettuce, roughly chopped
- 1 (15-ounce) can black beans, rinsed and drained
- 1 cup cherry tomatoes, halved
- 1 cup frozen (and thawed) or fresh corn kernels
- 1 avocado, peeled, pitted, and diced
- 4 scallions, thinly sliced

- 12 tortilla chips, crushed

Directions

1. To make the vinaigrette: In a small bowl, whisk together all the vinaigrette ingredients.
2. To make the salad: In a medium bowl, mix together the quinoa and taco seasoning. In a large bowl, toss the romaine with the vinaigrette. Divide among 4 bowls. Top each bowl with equal amounts quinoa, beans, tomatoes, corn, avocado, scallions, and crushed tortillas chips.

French-Style Potato Salad

Preparation Time: 5 Minutes

Cooking Time: 30 Minutes

Servings:4 To 6

Ingredients

- 11/2 pounds small white potatoes, unpeeled
- 2 tablespoons minced fresh parsley
- 1 tablespoon minced fresh chives
- 1 teaspoon minced fresh tarragon or 1/2 teaspoon dried
- 1/3 cup olive oil
- 2 tablespoons white wine or tarragon vinegar
- 1/8 teaspoon freshly ground black pepper

Directions

1. In a large pot of boiling salted water, cook the potatoes until tender but still firm, about 30 minutes.
2. Drain and cut into 1/4-inch slices. Transfer to a large bowl and add the parsley, chives, and tarragon.

3. Set aside.

4. In a small bowl, combine the oil, vinegar, pepper.

5. Pour the dressing onto the potato mixture and toss gently to combine.

6. Taste, adjusting seasonings if necessary.

7. Chill for 1 to 2 hours before serving.

Black Sesame Wonton Chips

Preparation time: 5 minutes

cooking time: 5 minutes

servings: 24 chips

Ingredients

- 12 Vegan Wonton Wrappers
- Toasted sesame oil
- 1/3 cup black sesame seeds
- Salt

Directions

1. Preheat the oven to 450°F. Lightly oil a baking sheet and set aside. Cut the wonton wrappers in half crosswise, brush them with sesame oil, and arrange them in a single layer on the prepared baking sheet.

2. Sprinkle wonton wrappers with the sesame seeds and salt to taste, and bake until crisp and golden brown, 5 to 7 minutes. Cool completely before serving. These are best eaten on the day they are made but, once cooled, they can be covered and stored at room temperature for 1 to 2 days.

Tempeh Tantrum Burgers

Preparation time: 15 minutes

cooking time: 0 minutes

servings: 4 burgers

Ingredients

- 8 ounces tempeh, cut into 1/2-inch dice
- ¾ cup chopped onion
- 2 garlic cloves, chopped
- ¾ cup chopped walnuts
- 1/2 cup old-fashioned or quick-cooking oats
- 1 tablespoon minced fresh parsley
- 1/2 teaspoon dried oregano
- 1/2 teaspoon dried thyme
- 1/2 teaspoon salt
- 1/4 teaspoon freshly ground black pepper
- 3 tablespoons olive oil
- Dijon mustard
- 4 whole grain burger rolls
- Sliced red onion, tomato, lettuce, and avocado

Directions

1. In a medium saucepan of simmering water, cook the tempeh for 30 minutes. Drain and set aside to cool.

2. In a food processor, combine the onion and garlic and process until minced. Add the cooled tempeh, the walnuts, oats, parsley, oregano, thyme, salt, and pepper. Process until well blended. Shape the mixture into 4 equal patties.

3. In a large skillet, heat the oil over medium heat. Add the burgers and cook until cooked thoroughly and browned on both sides, about 7 minutes per side.

4. Spread desired amount of mustard onto each half of the rolls and layer each roll with lettuce, tomato, red onion, and avocado, as desired. Serve immediately.

Keto Almond Zucchini Bread

Preparation Time: 15 minutes

Cooking Time: 35 minutes

Servings: 8

Ingredients:

- 2 eggs
- 1 c. zucchini, grated
- 1½ c. almond flour
- 1 c. chopped almonds
- ¾ c. Stevia
- 1 tbsp. ground cinnamon
- 1 tsp. pure vanilla extract
- 2 tbsps. coconut oil
- 1 tsp. baking soda
- Salt

Directions:

1. Preheat oven to 360F degrees.
2. Grease a loaf pan with melted coconut oil and set aside.

3. Whisk the eggs, organic vanilla extract, coconut oil and Stevia in a bowl.
4. With the help of an electric mixer, beat the egg mixture until combined well.
5. Add the almond flour, baking soda, salt and ground cinnamon and continue to mix.
6. Add in grated zucchini and chopped almonds and mix again until all ingredients combined well.
7. Pour the mixture in a prepared loaf pan and bake for 35 minutes.
8. Let cool for 10 minutes, slice and serve.

Nutrition:

Calories: 33, Fat: 7.27g, Carbs: 8.58g, Protein: 4.78g

Baked Onion Rings

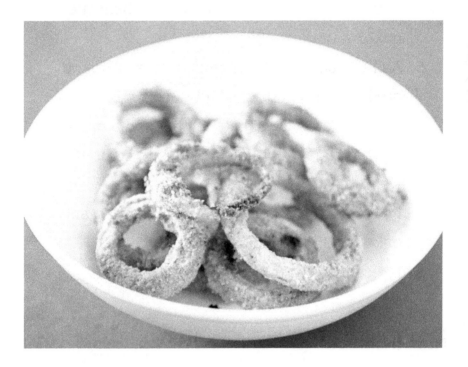

Preparation Time: 5 minutes

Cooking Time: 25 minutes

Servings: 4

Ingredients:

- 2 eggs, organic
- ½ teaspoon pepper
- ½ teaspoon salt

- ½ teaspoon garlic powder
- 2 tablespoons thyme, sliced
- 1 ½ cups almond flour
- 2 large sweet onions, cut into rings

Directions:

1. Preheat your oven to 400° Fahrenheit. In a mixing bowl, combine garlic powder, almond flour, thyme, garlic powder, and salt.
2. Take another bowl, add eggs and whisk. Dip the onion ring in egg mixture then coat with flour mixture.
3. Place the coated onion rings in a baking dish.
4. Bake in preheated oven for 25 minutes.
5. Serve immediately and enjoy!

Nutrition:

Calories: 130 Carbohydrates: 10.7 G Fat: 7.4 G
Sugar: 3.5 G Cholesterol: 82 Mg Protein: 6.1 G

Cheese Fries

Preparation Time: 5 minutes

Cooking Time: 4 minutes

Servings: 4

Ingredients:

- 8-ounces halloumi cheese, sliced into fries
- 2-ounces tallow
- 1 serving marinara sauce, low carb

Directions:

1. Heat the tallow in a pan over medium heat.
2. Gently place halloumi pieces in the pan.
3. Cook halloumi fries for 2 minutes on each side or until lightly golden brown.
4. Serve with marinara sauce and enjoy!

Nutrition:

Calories: 200 Sugar: 0.3 g Fat: 18 g Carbohydrates: 1 g Cholesterol: 42 mg Protein: 12 g

Roasted Cashews

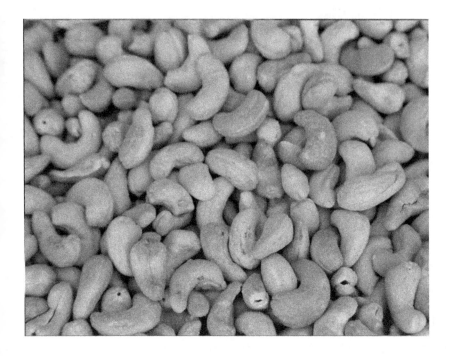

Preparation Time: 5 minutes

Cooking Time: 3 hours

Servings: 4

Ingredients:

- 1 cup cashews
- 1 cup water
- 2 tablespoons cinnamon

Directions:

1. Add water and cashews to a bowl and soak overnight.
2. Drain the cashews and place on a paper towel to dry.
3. Preheat oven to 200° Fahrenheit.
4. Place the soaked cashews on a baking tray.
5. Sprinkle cashews with cinnamon.
6. Roast in preheated oven for 3 hours.
7. Allow cooling time and then serve and enjoy!

Nutrition:

Calories: 205 Sugar: 1.8 g Fat: 15.9 g Carbohydrates: 13.9 g Cholesterol: 0 mg Protein: 5.4 g

Roasted Carrots

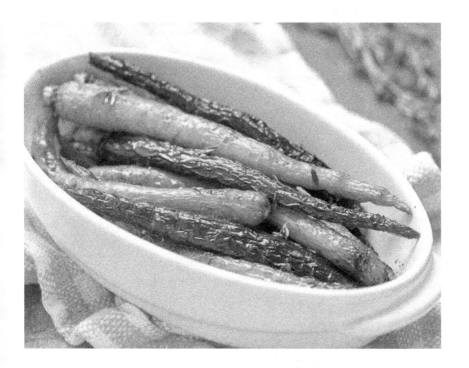

Preparation Time: 10 minutes

Cooking Time: 35 minutes

Servings: 6

Ingredients:

- 16 small carrots
- 1 tbsp fresh parsley, chopped
- 1 tbsp dried basil

- 6 garlic cloves, minced
- 4 tbsp olive oil
- 1 1/2 tsp salt

Directions:

1. Preheat the oven to 375 F/ 190 C.
2. In a bowl, combine together oil, carrots, basil, garlic, and salt.
3. Spread the carrots onto a baking tray and bake in preheated oven for 35 minutes.
4. Garnish with parsley and serve.

Nutrition:

Calories 139 Fat 9.4 g Carbohydrates 14.2 g Sugar 6.6 g Protein 1.3 g Cholesterol 0 mg

Smokey Cheddar Cheese (vegan)

Preparation time: 20 minutes

Cooking time: 0 minute

Servings: 8

Ingredients:

- 1 cup raw cashews (unsalted)
- 1 cup macadamia nuts (unsalted)
- 4 tsp. tapioca starch
- 1 cup water
- ¼ cup fresh lime juice
- ¼ cup tahini
- ½ tsp. liquid smoke
- ¼ cup paprika powder
- ½ tsp. ground mustard seeds
- 2 tbsp. onion powder
- 1 tsp. Himalayan salt
- ½ tsp. chili powder
- 1 tbsp. coconut oil

Directions:

1. Cover the cashews with water in a small bowl and let sit for 4 to 6 hours.
2. Rinse and drain the cashews after soaking.
3. Make sure no water is left.
4. Mix the tapioca starch with the cup of water in a small saucepan. Heat the pan over medium heat.
5. Bring the water with tapioca starch to a boil. After 1 minute, take the pan off the heat and set the mixture aside to cool down.
6. Put all the remaining ingredients—except the coconut oil—in a blender or food processor.
7. Blend until these ingredients are combined into a smooth mixture.
8. Stir in the tapioca starch with water and blend again until all ingredients have fully incorporated.
9. Grease a medium-sized bowl with the coconut oil to prevent the cheese from sticking to the edges.
10. Gently pour the mixture into the bowl.

11. Refrigerate the bowl, uncovered, for about 3 hours until the cheese is firm and ready to enjoy!
12. Alternatively, store the cheese in an airtight container in the fridge and consume within 6 days.
13. Store for a maximum of 60 days in the freezer and thaw at room temperature.

Nutrition:

Calories: 249 kcal, Net Carbs: 6.9g, Fat: 21.7g, Protein: 6.1g, Fiber: 4.3g, Sugar: 2.6g

Zucchini & Ricotta Tart

Preparation Time: 25 minutes

Cooking Time: about 1 hour

Servings: 8

Ingredients:

For the crust:

- 1¾ cups almond flour
- 1 tablespoon coconut flour
- ½ teaspoon garlic powder
- ¼ teaspoon salt
- ¼ cup melted butter

For the filling:

- 1 medium-large zucchini, thinly sliced cross-wise (use a mandolin if you have one)
- ½ teaspoon salt
- 8 ounces ricotta
- 3 large eggs
- ¼ cup whipping cream
- 2 cloves garlic, minced
- 1 teaspoon fresh dill, minced
- Additional salt and pepper to taste

- ½ cup shredded parmesan

Directions:

To make the crust:

1. Preheat oven to 325°F.
2. Lightly spray 9-inch ceramic or glass tart pan with cooking spray.
3. Combine the almond flour, coconut flour, garlic powder and salt in a large bowl.
4. Add the butter and stir until dough resembles coarse crumbs.
5. Press the dough gently into the tart pan, trimming away any excess.
6. Bake 15 minutes then remove from the oven and let cool.

To make the filling:

7. While crust is baking, put the zucchini slices into a colander and sprinkle each layer with a little salt. Let sit and drain for 30 minutes.
8. Place salted zucchini between double layers of paper towels and gently press down to remove any excess water.

9. Place the ricotta, eggs, whipping cream, garlic, dill, salt and pepper in a bowl and stir well to combine. Add almost all the zucchini slices, reserving about 25-30 for layering on top.
10. Transfer mixture into cooled crust. Top with the remaining zucchini slices, slightly overlapping.
11. Sprinkle with parmesan cheese.
12. Bake 60 to 70 minutes or until center is no longer wobbly and a toothpick comes out clean.
13. Cut into slices and serve.

Nutrition:

Calories: 302, Total Fats: 25.2g, Carbohydrates: 7.9g, Fiber: 3.1g, Protein: 12.4g

Minty Fruit Salad

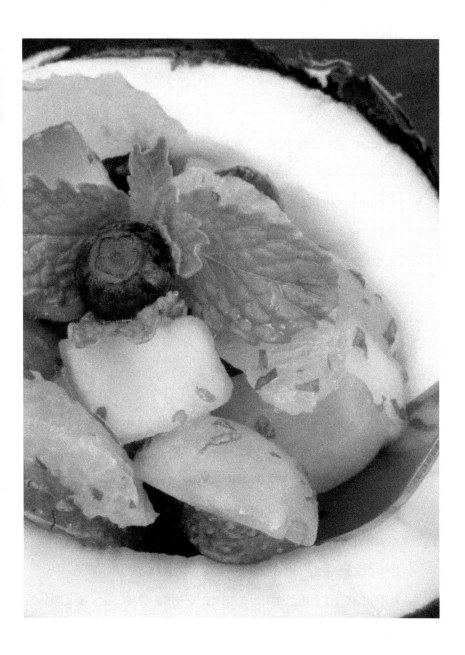

Preparation time: 15 minutes

cooking time: 5 minutes

servings: 4

Ingredients

- ¼ cup lemon juice (about 2 small lemons
- 4 teaspoons maple syrup or agave syrup
- 2 cups chopped pineapple
- 2 cups chopped strawberries
- 2 cups raspberries
- 1 cup blueberries
- 8 fresh mint leaves

Directions

1. Beginning with 1 mason jar, add the ingredients in this order:
2. 1 tablespoon of lemon juice, 1 teaspoon of maple syrup, ½ cup of pineapple, ½ cup of strawberries, ½ cup of raspberries, ¼ cup of blueberries, and 2 mint leaves.
3. Repeat to fill 3 more jars. Close the jars tightly with lids.

4. Place the airtight jars in the refrigerator for up to 3 days.

Nutrition:

Calories: 138; Fat: 1g; Protein: 2g; Carbohydrates: 34g; Fiber: 8g; Sugar: 22g; Sodium: 6mg

Coconut and Almond Truffles

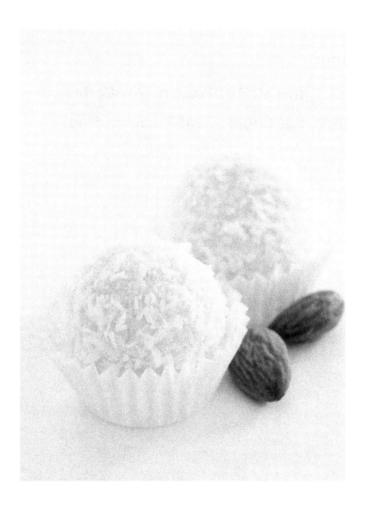

Preparation time: 15 minutes

cooking time: 0 minutes

servings: 8 truffles

Ingredients

- 1 cup pitted dates
- 1 cup almonds
- ½ cup sweetened cocoa powder, plus extra for coating
- ½ cup unsweetened shredded coconut
- ¼ cup pure maple syrup
- 1 teaspoon vanilla extract
- 1 teaspoon almond extract
- ¼ teaspoon sea salt

Directions

1. In the bowl of a food processor, combine all the ingredients and process until smooth. Chill the mixture for about 1 hour.
2. Roll the mixture into balls and then roll the balls in cocoa powder to coat.
3. Serve immediately or keep chilled until ready to serve.

Fruits Stew

Preparation time: 10 minutes

Cooking time: 10 minutes

Servings: 4

Ingredients:

- 1 avocado, peeled, pitted and sliced
- 1 cup plums, stoned and halved
- 2 cups water
- 2 teaspoons vanilla extract
- 1 tablespoon lemon juice
- 2 tablespoons stevia

Directions:

1. In a pan, combine the avocado with the plums, water and the other ingredients, bring to a simmer and cook over medium heat for 10 minutes.
2. Divide the mix into bowls and serve cold.

Nutrition:

calories 178, fat 4.4, fiber 2, carbs 3, protein 5

Ginger Cream

Preparation time: 10 minutes

Cooking time: 10 minutes

Servings: 4

Ingredients:

- 2 tablespoons stevia
- 2 cups coconut cream
- 1 teaspoon vanilla extract
- 1 tablespoon cinnamon powder
- ¼ tablespoon ginger, grated

Directions:

1. In a pan, combine the cream with the stevia and other ingredients, stir, cook over medium heat for 10 minutes, divide into bowls and serve cold.

Nutrition:

calories 280, fat 28.6, fiber 2.7, carbs 7, protein 2.8

Cream Cheese Frosting.

Preparation Time: 5 Minutes

Servings: 2.5 cups

Ingredients:

- 1½ cups confectioners' sugar
- 1 cup vegan cream cheese at room temperature
- ½ cup vegan butter, at room temperature
- 1 teaspoon pure vanilla extract

Directions:

1. Combine all the ingredients until smoothly blended.

Orange Polenta Cake.

Preparation Time: 30 Minutes

Servings: 6

Ingredients:

- 1¼ cups all-purpose flour
- 1 cup unsweetened almond milk
- 2/3 cup plus 1 tablespoon natural sugar
- ⅓ cup fine-ground cornmeal
- ⅓ cup plus 2 tablespoons marmalade
- ¼ cup finely ground almonds
- ¼ cup vegan butter, softened
- 1 navel orange, peeled and sliced into ⅛-inch-thick rounds
- 1½ teaspoons baking powder
- 1 teaspoon pure vanilla extract
- ¾ teaspoon salt

Directions:

1. Lightly oil a baking tray that will fit in the steamer basket of your Cooker.

2. Sprinkle a tablespoon of sugar over the base of the baking tray and top with the orange slices.

3. In a bowl combine the flour, cornmeal, baking powder, almonds, and salt.

4. In another bowl combine the remaining sugar, the butter, 1/3 cup of marmalade, and vanilla and mix well. Slowly stir in the almond milk.

5. Combine the wet and dry mixes into a smooth batter.

6. Pour the batter into your baking tray and put the tray in your steamer basket.

7. Pour the minimum amount of water into the base of your Cooker and lower the steamer basket.

8. Seal and cook on Steam for 12 minutes.

9. Release the pressure quickly and set to one side to cool a little.

10. Warm the remaining 2 tablespoons of marmalade and brush over the cake.

Peanut Butter & Chocolate Cheesecake.

Preparation Time: 30 Minutes

Servings: 8

Ingredients:

- 16 ounces vegan cream cheese
- 8 ounces silken tofu, drained
- 1½ cups crushed vegan chocolate cookies
- ¾ cup natural sugar
- ½ cup creamy peanut butter, at room temperature
- ¼ cup unsweetened cocoa powder
- 3 tablespoons vegan butter, melted
- 2 tablespoons hazelnut milk

Directions:

1. Lightly oil a baking tray that will fit in the steamer basket of your Cooker.
2. Combine the chocolate crumbs and the butter.
3. Press the chocolate base into your tray.
4. Blend the cream cheese and tofu until smooth.

5. Add the peanut butter, cocoa, hazelnut milk, and sugar to the cheese mix and fold in well.

6. Pour the cheese onto your base and put the tray in your steamer basket.

7. Pour the minimum amount of water into the base of your Cooker and lower the steamer basket.

8. Seal and cook on Steam for 15 minutes.

9. Release the pressure quickly and set to one side to cool a little.

Grapes Vanilla Cream

Preparation time: 1 hour

Cooking time: 0 minutes

Servings: 4

Ingredients:

- 2 cups almond milk
- 1 cup grapes, halved
- 1 cup coconut cream
- 3 tablespoons stevia
- 1 teaspoon vanilla extract
- 1 teaspoon gelatin powder

Directions:

1. In a bowl, combine the grapes with the coconut cream, the almond milk and the other ingredients, whisk well, divide into cups and keep in the fridge for 1 hour before serving.

Nutrition:

calories 432, fat 43, fiber 4.2, carbs 14, protein 4.3

Cold Grapes and Avocado Cream

Preparation time: 1 hour

Cooking time: 0 minutes

Servings: 4

Ingredients:

- ½ cup stevia
- 2 cups grapes, halved
- 1 avocado, peeled, pitted and chopped
- 1 cup almond milk
- Zest of 1 lime, grated
- ½ cup coconut cream

Directions:

1. In a blender, combine the grapes with the avocado and the other ingredients, pulse well, divide into bowls and keep in the fridge for 1 hour before serving.

Nutrition:

calories 152, fat 4.4, fiber 5.5, carbs 5.1, protein 0.8

NOTE

CPSIA information can be obtained
at www.ICGtesting.com
Printed in the USA
BVHW040824290621
610724BV00017B/479

9 781801 93072